EASY DASH DIET RECIPES

The Every Day Dash Diet Cookbook. Fresh and Delicious Recipes for Beginners to Speed Weigh Loss, Lower Blood Pressure and Prevent Diabetes.

Victoria Green

Table of Contents:

GREAT DASH DIET RECIPES

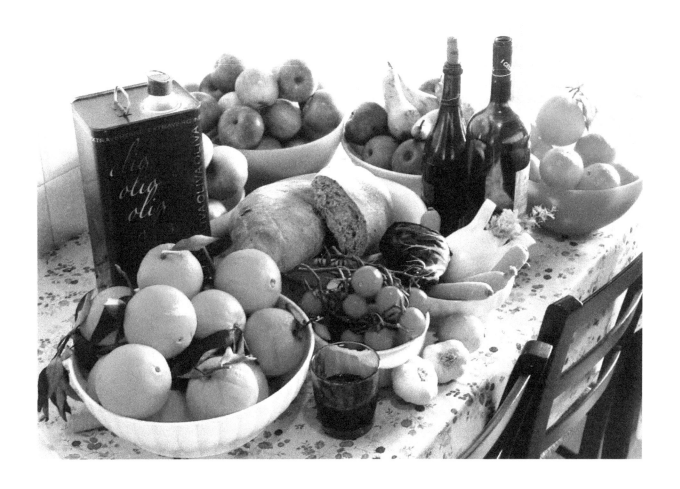

Spiced Chicken-stuffed Zucchini With Brown Rice And Lentils

Servings: 3

Cooking Time: 35 Minutes

Ingredients:

⅓ cup long-grain brown rice

1⅔ cups water

⅛ teaspoon kosher salt

⅓ cup brown lentils

2 teaspoons olive oil

3 tablespoons chopped fresh dill

3 medium zucchini, halved lengthwise and flesh scooped out with a teaspoon (zucchini flesh reserved)

3 teaspoons olive oil, divided

1 small yellow onion, chopped

1 teaspoon chopped garlic

½ pound ground lean chicken

¾ teaspoon ground cumin

¾ teaspoon ground coriander

¾ teaspoon caraway seeds

⅛ teaspoon red chili flakes

3 tablespoons tomato paste

¼ teaspoon kosher salt

¼ cup feta cheese

Directions:

TO MAKE THE BROWN RICE AND LENTILS

Place the rice, water, and salt in a saucepan over high heat. Once the water is boiling, cover the pan and reduce the heat to low. Simmer for 15 minutes.

After 15 minutes, add the lentils and stir. Cover the pan and cook for another 15 minutes.

If there is a little bit of water still in the pan after the rice and lentils are tender, cook uncovered for a couple of minutes.

Stir in the oil and chopped dill.

Once the mixture has cooled, place ⅔ cup in each of 3 containers.

TO MAKE THE STUFFED ZUCCHINI

Preheat the oven to 400°F and line a sheet pan with a silicone baking mat or parchment paper. Place the zucchini boats on a lined sheet pan and coat with 1 teaspoon of oil.

In a 12-inch skillet, heat the remaining 2 teaspoons of oil over medium-high heat. When the oil is shimmering, add the onion and garlic and cook for 5 minutes. Add the zucchini flesh and cook for 2 more minutes.

Add the ground chicken, breaking it up with a spatula. Cook for 5 more minutes.

Add the cumin, coriander, caraway seeds, chili flakes, tomato paste, and salt, and cook for another 2 minutes.

Mound the chicken mixture into the zucchini boats. Top each zucchini boat with 2 teaspoons of feta cheese. Bake for 20 minutes.

Once cooled, place 2 zucchini halves in each of the 3 rice-and-lentil containers.

STORAGE: Store covered containers in the refrigerator for up to 5 days. Brown rice and lentils can be frozen for up to 3 months.

Nutrition Info: Total calories: 414; Total fat: 19g; Saturated fat: 5g; Sodium: 645mg; Carbohydrates: 39g; Fiber: 10g; Protein: 26g

Apple, Cinnamon, And Walnut Baked Oatmeal

Servings: 8

Cooking Time: 40 Minutes

Ingredients:

Cooking spray or oil for greasing the pan

3 small Granny Smith apples (about 1 pound), skin-on, chopped into ½-inch dice

3 cups rolled oats

1 teaspoon baking powder

3 tablespoons ground flaxseed

1 teaspoon ground cinnamon

2 eggs

¼ cup olive oil

1½ cups low-fat (2%) milk

⅓ cup pure maple syrup

½ cup walnut pieces (if you buy walnut halves, roughly chop the nuts)

Directions:

Preheat the oven to 350°F and spray an 8-by--inch baking dish with cooking spray or rub with oil.

Combine the apples, oats, baking powder, flaxseed, cinnamon, eggs, oil, milk, and maple syrup in a large mixing bowl and pour into the prepared baking dish.

Sprinkle the walnut pieces evenly across the oatmeal and bake for 40 minutes.

Allow the oatmeal to cool and cut it into 8 pieces. Place 1 piece in each of 5 containers. Take the other 3 pieces and either eat as a snack during the week or freeze for a later time.

STORAGE: Store covered containers in the refrigerator for up to 6 days. If frozen, oatmeal will last 6 months.

Nutrition Info: Total calories: 349; Total fat: 18g; Saturated fat: 3g; Sodium: 108mg; Carbohydrates: 43g; Fiber: ; Protein: 9g

Chocolate–peanut Butter Yogurt With Berries

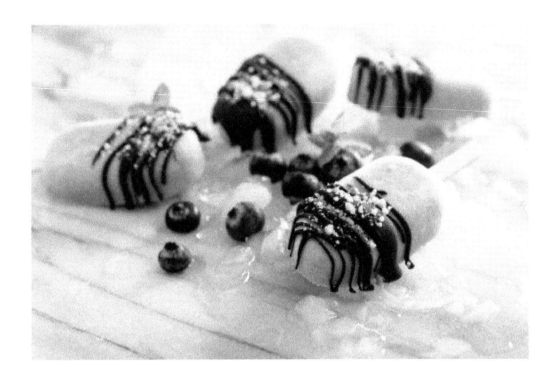

Servings: 4

Cooking Time: 15 Minutes

Ingredients:

2 cups low-fat (2%) plain Greek yogurt

4 tablespoons unsweetened cocoa powder

4 tablespoons natural-style peanut butter

1 tablespoon pure maple syrup

1 cup fresh or frozen berries of your choice

Directions:

In a medium bowl, mix the yogurt, cocoa powder, peanut butter, and maple syrup until well combined.

Spoon ½ cup of the yogurt mixture and ¼ cup of berries into each of 4 containers.

STORAGE: Store covered containers in the refrigerator for up to 5 days.

Nutrition Info: Total calories: 225; Total fat: 12g; Saturated fat: ; Sodium: 130mg; Carbohydrates: 19g; Fiber: 4g; Protein: 16g

Olive Fougasse

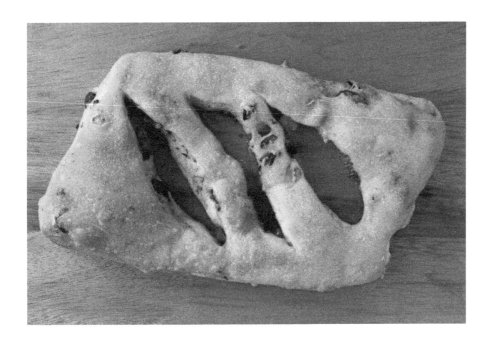

Servings: 4

Cooking Time: 20 Minutes

Ingredients:

3 2/3 cups bread flour

3 1/2 tablespoons olive oil

1 2/3 tablespoons bread yeast

1 1/4 cups black olives, chopped

1 teaspoon oregano

1 teaspoon salt

1 cup water

Directions:

Add flour to a bowl.

Make a well in the center and add the water and remaining Ingredients:.

Knead the dough well until it becomes slightly elastic.

Mold it into a ball and let stand for about 1 hour.

Divide the pastry into four pieces of equal portions.

Flatten the balls using a rolling pin and place it on a floured baking tray.

Make incisions on the bread.

Allow them to rest for about 30 minutes

Preheat oven to 425 degrees Fahrenheit.

Brush the Fougasse with olive oil and allow it to bake for 20 minutes.

Turn the oven off and allow it to rest for 5 minutes.

Remove and allow it to cool.

Enjoy!

Nutrition Info: Calories: 586, Total Fat: 18.1 g, Saturated Fat: 2.6 g, Cholesterol: 0 mg, Sodium: 371 mg, Total Carbohydrate: 92.2 g, Dietary Fiber: 5.6 g, Total Sugars: 0.3 g, Protein: 2 g, Vitamin D: 0 mcg, Calcium: 63 mg, Iron: 8 mg, Potassium: 232 mg

Tofu And Vegetable Provençal

Servings: 4

Cooking Time: 30 Minutes

Ingredients:

1 pound super-firm tofu, cut into ¾-inch cubes

2 tablespoons freshly squeezed lemon juice

2 tablespoons olive oil

1 teaspoon garlic powder

1 teaspoon herbes de Provence

¼ teaspoon kosher salt

4 teaspoons olive oil, divided

1 (14-ounce) eggplant, cubed into 1-inch pieces (5 to 6 cups)

1 small yellow onion, chopped (about 2 cups)

2 teaspoons chopped garlic

10 ounces cherry tomatoes, halved if tomatoes are fairly large

1 (14-ounce) can artichoke hearts, drained

1 teaspoon herbes de Provence

¼ teaspoon kosher salt

½ cup dry white wine, such as sauvignon blanc

⅓ cup pitted kalamata olives, roughly chopped

1 (½-ounce) package fresh basil, chopped

Directions:

TO MAKE THE TOFU

Place the tofu in a container with the lemon juice, oil, garlic powder, herbes de Provence, and salt. Allow to marinate for 1 hour.

When you're ready to cook the tofu, preheat the oven to 400°F and line a sheet pan with a silicone baking mat or parchment paper. Lift the tofu out of the marinade and place it on the sheet pan. Bake for minutes, flipping the tofu over after 15 minutes. Cool, then place about ½ cup of tofu cubes in each of 4 containers.

TO MAKE THE VEGETABLE RAGOUT

While the tofu is marinating, heat 2 teaspoons of oil in a 12-inch skillet over medium-high heat. When the oil is shimmering, add the eggplant and cook for 4 minutes, stirring occasionally. Remove the eggplant and place on a plate.

Add the remaining 2 teaspoons of oil to the pan, and add the onion and garlic. Cook for 2 minutes. Add the tomatoes and cook for 5 more minutes. Add the eggplant, artichokes, herbes de Provence, salt, and wine. Cover the pan, lower the heat, and simmer for 20 minutes.

Turn the heat off and stir in the olives and basil.

Spoon about 1½ cups of vegetables into each of the 4 tofu containers.

STORAGE: Store covered containers in the refrigerator for up to 5 days.

Nutrition Info: Total calories: 362; Total fat: 17g; Saturated fat: 3g; Sodium: 728mg; Carbohydrates: 32g; Fiber: 9g; Protein: 23g

Banana, Orange, And Pistachio Smoothie

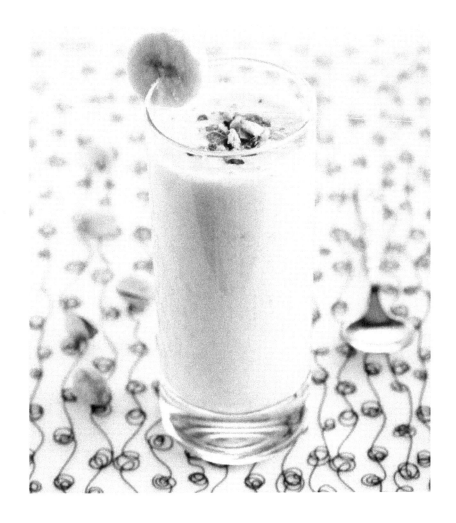

Servings: 3

Cooking Time: 25 Minutes

Ingredients:

1 (17.6-ounce) container plain low-fat (2%) Greek yogurt

3 very ripe medium bananas

1½ cups orange juice

¾ cup unsalted shelled pistachios

Directions:

Place all the ingredients in a blender and blend until smooth.

Pour 1¾ cups of the smoothie into each of 3 smoothie containers.

STORAGE: Store covered containers in the refrigerator for up to 4 days.

Nutrition Info: calories: 9; Total fat: 19g; Saturated fat: 4g; Sodium: 71mg; Carbohydrates: 55g; Fiber: 3g; Protein: 26g

Breakfast Bento Box

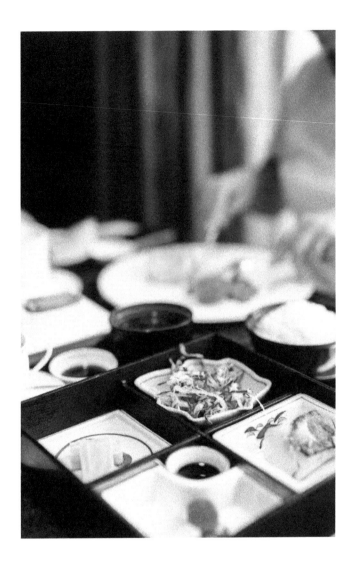

Servings: 2

Cooking Time: 12 Minutes

Ingredients:

2 eggs

2 ounces sliced prosciutto

20 small whole-grain crackers

20 whole, unsalted almonds (about ¼ cup)

2 (6-inch) Persian cucumbers, sliced

1 large pear, sliced

Directions:

Place the eggs in a saucepan and cover with water. Bring the water to a boil. As soon as the water starts to boil, place a lid on the pan and turn the heat off. Set a timer for minutes.

When the timer goes off, drain the hot water and run cold water over the eggs to cool. Peel the eggs when cool and cut in half.

Place 2 egg halves and half of the prosciutto, crackers, almonds, cucumber slices, and pear slices in each of 2 containers.

STORAGE: Store covered containers in the refrigerator for up to 5 days.

Nutrition Info: Total calories: 370; Total fat: 20g; Saturated fat: ; Sodium: 941mg; Carbohydrates: 35g; Fiber: 7g; Protein: 16g

Maple-cardamom Chia Pudding With Blueberries

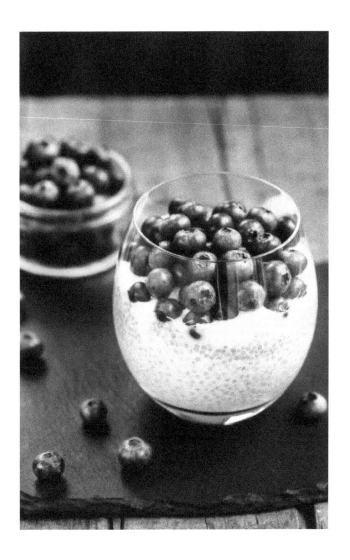

Servings: 5

Cooking Time: 5 Minutes

Ingredients:

2½ cups low-fat (2%) milk

½ cup chia seeds

1 tablespoon plus 1 teaspoon pure maple syrup

¼ teaspoon ground cardamom

2½ cups frozen blueberries

Directions:

Place the milk, chia seeds, maple syrup, and cardamom in a large bowl and stir to combine.

Spoon ½ cup of the mixture into each of 5 containers.

Place ½ cup of frozen blueberries in each container and stir to combine. Let the pudding sit for at least an hour in the refrigerator before eating.

STORAGE: Store covered containers in the refrigerator for up to 5 days.

Nutrition Info: Total calories: 218; Total fat: 8g; Saturated fat: 2g; Sodium: 74mg; Carbohydrates: 28g; Fiber: 10g; Protein: 10g

Cheesy Bread

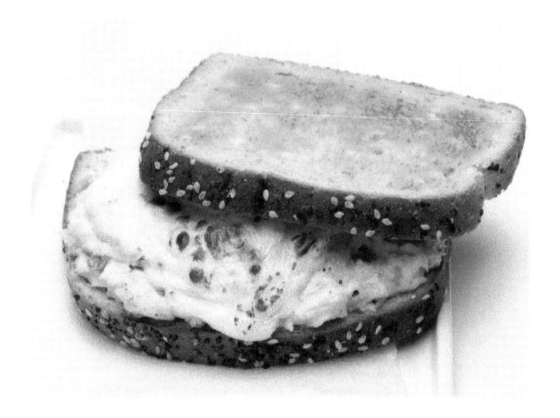

Servings: 12

Cooking Time: 15 Minutes

Ingredients:

3 cups shredded cheddar cheese

1 cup mayonnaise

1 1-ounce pack dry ranch dressing mix

1 2-ounce can chopped black olives, drained

4 green onions, sliced

2 French baguettes, cut into ½ inch slices

Directions:

Preheat oven to 350 degrees Fahrenheit.

In a medium-sized bowl, combine cheese, ranch dressing mix, mayonnaise, onions, and olives.

Increase mayo if you want a juicier mixture.

Spread cheese mixture on top of your French baguette slices.

Arrange the slices in a single layer on a large baking sheet.

Bake for about 15 minutes until the cheese is bubbly and browning.

Cool and chill.

Serve warm!

Nutrition Info: Calories: 2, Total Fat: 17 g, Saturated Fat: 7.2 g, Cholesterol: 35 mg, Sodium: 578 mg, Total Carbohydrate: 23.9 g, Dietary Fiber: 1.1 g, Total Sugars: 2.4 g, Protein: 11.1 g, Vitamin D: 3 mcg, Calcium: 229 mg, Iron: 2 mg, Potassium: 85 mg

Carrot-chickpea Fritters

Servings: 3

Cooking Time: 10 Minutes

Ingredients:

2 teaspoons olive oil, plus 1 tablespoon

3 cups shredded carrots

1 (4-ounce) bunch scallions, white and green parts chopped

1 (15-ounce) can low-sodium chickpeas, drained and rinsed

⅓ cup dried apricots (about 10 small apricot halves), chopped

1 teaspoon garlic powder

1½ teaspoons dried mint

⅓ cup chickpea flour

1 egg

¼ teaspoon kosher salt

1 tablespoon freshly squeezed lemon juice

1 (5-ounce) package arugula

¾ cup Garlic Yogurt Sauce

Directions:

Heat 2 teaspoons of oil in a -inch skillet over medium-high heat. Once the oil is hot, add the carrots and scallions, and cook for 5 minutes. Allow to cool.

While the carrots are cooking, mash the chickpeas in a large mixing bowl with the bottom of a coffee mug. (I find a coffee mug works better than a potato masher.)

Add the apricots, garlic powder, mint, chickpea flour, egg, salt, lemon juice, and cooked carrot mixture to the bowl, and stir until well combined.

Form 6 patties and place them on a plate.

Heat the remaining 1 tablespoon of oil in the same skillet over medium-high heat. Once the oil is hot, add the patties. Cook for 3 minutes on each side, or until each side is browned.

Place 2 cooled fritters in each of 3 containers. Place about 2 cups of arugula in each of 3 other containers, and spoon ¼ cup Garlic Yogurt Sauce into each of 3 separate containers, or next to the arugula. The arugula and sauce are served at room temperature, while the fritters will be reheated.

STORAGE:Store covered containers in the refrigerator for up to 5 days. Uncooked patties can be frozen for 3 to 4 months.

Nutrition Info: Total calories: 461; Total fat: 17g; Saturated fat: 3g; Sodium: 393mg; Carbohydrates: 61g; Fiber: 15g; Protein: 21g

Whole-wheat Pasta With Lentil Bolognese

Servings: 4

Cooking Time: 55 Minutes

Ingredients:

2 tablespoons olive oil, divided

1 small yellow onion, chopped (about 2 cups)

1 tablespoon chopped garlic

2 medium carrots, peeled, halved vertically, and sliced (about 1¼ cup)

8 ounces button or cremini mushrooms, roughly chopped (about 4 cups)

1 teaspoon dried Italian herbs

2 tablespoons tomato paste

½ cup dry red wine

1 (28-ounce) can no-salt-added crushed tomatoes

2 cups water

1 cup uncooked brown lentils

½ teaspoon kosher salt

8 ounces dry whole-wheat penne pasta

¼ cup nutritional yeast

Directions:

Heat a soup pot on medium-high heat with tablespoon of oil. Once the oil is shimmering, add the onion and garlic, and cook for 2 minutes.

Add the carrots and mushrooms, then stir and cook for another 5 minutes.

Add the Italian herbs and tomato paste, stir to evenly incorporate, and cook for 5 more minutes, without stirring.

Add the wine and scrape up any bits from the bottom of the pan. Cook for 2 more minutes.

Add the tomatoes, water, lentils, and salt. Bring to a boil, then turn the heat down to low and simmer for 40 minutes.

While the sauce is cooking, cook the pasta according to the package directions, drain, and cool.

When the sauce is done simmering, stir in the remaining 1 tablespoon of oil and the nutritional yeast. Cool the sauce.

Combine 1 cup of cooked pasta and 1⅓ cups of sauce in each of 4 containers. Freeze the remaining sauce for a later meal.

STORAGE: Store covered containers in the refrigerator for up to 5 days.

Nutrition Info: Total calories: 570; Total fat: 9g; Saturated fat: 1g; Sodium: 435mg; Carbohydrates: 96g; Fiber: 17g; Protein: 27g

Strawberries With Cottage Cheese And Pistachios

Servings: 5

Cooking Time: 35 Minutes

Ingredients:

16 ounces low-fat cottage cheese

16 ounces strawberries, hulled and sliced

½ cup plus 2 tablespoons unsalted shelled pistachios

Directions:

Spoon ⅓ cup of cottage cheese into each of 5 containers.

Top each scoop of cottage cheese with ⅔ cup of strawberries and tablespoons of pistachios.

Refrigerate.

STORAGE: Store covered containers in the refrigerator for up to 5 days.

Nutrition Info: Total calories: 184; Total fat: 9g; Saturated fat: 2g; Sodium: 26g; Carbohydrates: 14g; Fiber: 4g; Protein: 15g

Turkey Meatballs With Tomato Sauce And Roasted Spaghetti Squash

Servings: 3

Cooking Time: 35 Minutes

Ingredients:

FOR THE SPAGHETTI SQUASH

3 pounds spaghetti squash

1 teaspoon olive oil

¼ teaspoon kosher salt

FOR THE MEATBALLS

½ pound lean ground turkey

4 ounces mushrooms, finely chopped (about 1½ cups)

2 tablespoons onion powder

1 tablespoon garlic powder

1 teaspoon dried Italian herbs

⅛ teaspoon kosher salt

1 large egg

FOR THE SAUCE

1 (28-ounce) can crushed tomatoes

1 cup shredded carrots

1 teaspoon garlic powder

1 teaspoon onion powder

¼ teaspoon kosher salt

Directions:

TO MAKE THE SPAGHETTI SQUASH

Preheat the oven to 4°F and place a silicone baking mat or parchment paper on a sheet pan.

Using a heavy, sharp knife, cut the ends off the spaghetti squash. Stand the squash upright and cut down the middle. Scrape out the seeds and stringy flesh with a spoon and discard.

Rub the oil on the cut sides of the squash and sprinkle with the salt. Lay the squash cut-side down on the baking sheet. Roast for 30 to 35 minutes, until the flesh is tender when poked with a sharp knife.

When the squash is cool enough to handle, scrape the flesh out with a fork and place about 1 cup in each of 3 containers.

TO MAKE THE MEATBALLS AND SAUCE

Place all the ingredients for the meatballs in a large bowl. Mix with your hands until all the ingredients are combined.

Place all the sauce ingredients in an by-11-inch glass or ceramic baking dish, and stir to combine.

Form 12 golf-ball-size meatballs and place each directly in the baking dish of tomato sauce.

Place the baking dish in the oven and bake for 25 minutes. Cool.

Place 4 meatballs and 1 cup of sauce in each of the 3 squash containers.

STORAGE:Store covered containers in the refrigerator for up to 5 days.

Nutrition Info: Total calories: 406; Total fat: ; Saturated fat: 5g; Sodium: 1,296mg; Carbohydrates: 45g; Fiber: 10g; Protein: 29g

Salmon Cakes With Steamed Green Bean Gremolata

Servings: 4

Cooking Time: 6 Minutes

Ingredients:

2 (6-ounce) cans skinless, boneless salmon, drained

½ teaspoon garlic powder

⅓ cup minced shallot

2 tablespoons Dijon mustard

2 eggs

½ cup panko bread crumbs

1 tablespoon capers, chopped

1 cup chopped parsley

⅓ cup chopped sun-dried tomatoes

1 tablespoon freshly squeezed lemon juice

1 tablespoon olive oil

Zest of 2 lemons (about 2 tablespoons when zested with a Microplane)

¼ cup minced parsley

1 teaspoon minced garlic

¼ teaspoon kosher salt

1 teaspoon olive oil

1 pound green beans, trimmed

Directions:

TO MAKE THE SALMON CAKES

In a large bowl, place the salmon, garlic, shallot, mustard, eggs, bread crumbs, capers, parsley, tomatoes, and lemon juice. Stir well to combine.

Form 8 patties and place them on a plate.

Heat the oil in a 12-inch skillet over medium-high heat. Once the oil is hot, add the patties. Cook for 3 minutes on each side, or until each side is browned.

Place 2 cooled salmon cakes in each of 4 containers.

TO MAKE THE GREEN BEANS

In a small bowl, combine the lemon zest, parsley, garlic, salt, and oil.

Bring about ¼ to ½ inch of water to a boil in a soup pot, Dutch oven, or skillet.

Once the water is boiling, add the green beans, cover, and set a timer for 3 minutes. The green beans should be crisp-tender.

Drain the green beans and transfer to a large bowl. Add the gremolata (lemon zest mixture) and toss to combine.

Divide the green beans among the 4 salmon cake containers. If using, place ¼ cup of Garlic Yogurt Sauce in each of 4 sauce containers. Refrigerate.

STORAGE: Store covered containers in the refrigerator for up to 5 days. Uncooked patties can be frozen for 3 to 4 months.

Nutrition Info: Total calories: 268; Total fat: 9g; Saturated fat: 2g; Sodium: 638mg; Carbohydrates: 21g; Fiber: 6g; Protein: 27g

Popcorn Trail Mix

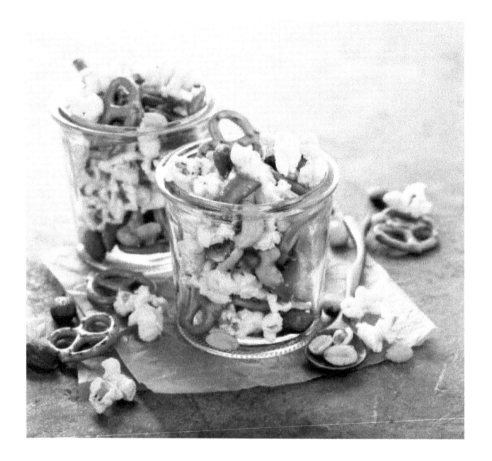

Servings: 5

Cooking Time: 35 Minutes

Ingredients:

12 dried apricot halves, quartered

⅔ cup whole, unsalted almonds

½ cup green pumpkin seeds (pepitas)

4 cups air-popped lightly salted popcorn

Directions:

Place the apricots, almonds, and pumpkin seeds in a medium bowl and toss with clean hands to evenly mix.

Scoop about ⅓ cup of the mixture into each of 5 containers or resealable sandwich bags. Place ¾ cup of popcorn in each of 5 separate containers or resealable bags. You will have one extra serving.

Mix the popcorn and the almond mixture together when it's time to eat. (The apricots make the popcorn stale quickly, which is why they're stored separately.)

STORAGE: Store covered containers or resealable bags at room temperature for up to 5 days.

Nutrition Info: Total calories: 244; Total fat: 16g; Saturated fat: 2g; Sodium: 48mg; Carbohydrates: 19g; Fiber: ; Protein: 10g

Creamy Shrimp-stuffed Portobello Mushrooms

Servings: 3

Cooking Time: 40 Minutes

Ingredients:

1 teaspoon olive oil, plus 2 tablespoons

6 portobello mushrooms, caps and stems separated and stems chopped

6 ounces broccoli florets, finely chopped (about 2 cups)

2 teaspoons chopped garlic

10 ounces uncooked peeled, deveined shrimp, thawed if frozen, roughly chopped

1 (14.5-ounce) can no-salt-added diced tomatoes

4 tablespoons roughly chopped fresh basil

½ cup mascarpone cheese

¼ cup panko bread crumbs

4 tablespoons grated Parmesan, divided

¼ teaspoon kosher salt

Directions:

Preheat the oven to 350°F. Line a sheet pan with a silicone baking mat or parchment paper.

Rub 1 teaspoon of oil over the bottom (stem side) of the mushroom caps and place on the lined sheet pan, stem-side up.

Heat the remaining 2 tablespoons of oil in a 12-inch skillet on medium-high heat. Once the oil is shimmering, add the chopped mushroom stems and broccoli, and sauté for 2 to minutes. Add the garlic and shrimp, and continue cooking for 2 more minutes.

Add the tomatoes, basil, mascarpone, bread crumbs, 3 tablespoons of Parmesan, and the salt. Stir to combine and turn the heat off.

With the mushroom cap openings facing up, mound slightly less than 1 cup of filling into each mushroom. Top each with ½ teaspoon of the remaining Parmesan cheese.

Bake the mushrooms for 35 minutes.

Place 2 mushroom caps in each of 3 containers.

STORAGE: Store covered containers in the refrigerator for up to 4 days.

Nutrition Info: Total calories: 47 Total fat: 31g; Saturated fat: 10g; Sodium: 526mg; Carbohydrates: 26g; Fiber: 7g; Protein: 26g

Rosemary Edamame, Zucchini, And Sun-dried Tomatoes With Garlic-chive Quinoa

Servings: 4

Cooking Time: 15 Minutes

Ingredients:

FOR THE GARLIC-CHIVE QUINOA

1 teaspoon olive oil

1 teaspoon chopped garlic

⅔ cup quinoa

1⅓ cups water

¼ teaspoon kosher salt

1 (¾-ounce) package fresh chives, chopped

FOR THE ROSEMARY EDAMAME, ZUCCHINI, AND SUN-DRIED TOMATOES

1 teaspoon oil from sun-dried tomato jar

2 medium zucchini, cut in half lengthwise and sliced into half-moons (about 3 cups)

1 (12-ounce) package frozen shelled edamame, thawed (2 cups)

½ cup julienne-sliced sun-dried tomatoes in olive oil, drained

¼ teaspoon dried rosemary

⅛ teaspoon kosher salt

Directions:

TO MAKE THE GARLIC-CHIVE QUINOA

Heat the oil over medium heat in a saucepan. Once the oil is shimmering, add the garlic and cook for 1 minute, stirring often so it doesn't burn.

Add the quinoa and stir a few times. Add the water and salt and turn the heat up to high. Once the water is boiling, cover the pan and turn the heat down to low. Simmer the quinoa for 15 minutes, or until the water is absorbed.

Stir in the chives and fluff the quinoa with a fork.

Place ½ cup quinoa in each of 4 containers.

TO MAKE THE ROSEMARY EDAMAME, ZUCCHINI, AND SUN-DRIED TOMATOES

Heat the oil in a 12-inch skillet over medium-high heat. Once the oil is shimmering, add the zucchini and cook for 2 minutes.

Add the edamame, sun-dried tomatoes, rosemary, and salt, and cook for another 6 minutes, or until the zucchini is crisp-tender.

Spoon 1 cup of the edamame mixture into each of the 4 quinoa containers.

STORAGE: Store covered containers in the refrigerator for up to 5 days.

Nutrition Info: Total calories: 312; Total fat: ; Saturated fat: 1g; Sodium: 389mg; Carbohydrates: 39g; Fiber: 9g; Protein: 15g

Cherry, Vanilla, And Almond Overnight Oats

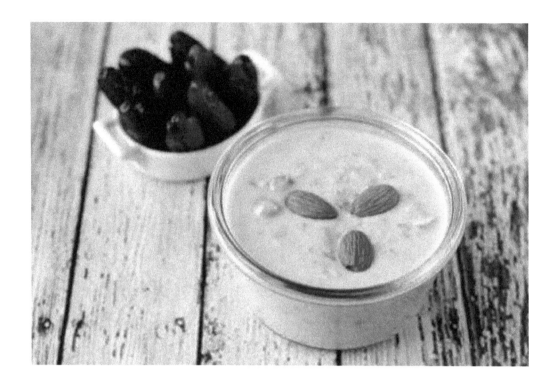

Servings: 5

Cooking Time: 10 Minutes

Ingredients:

1⅔ cups rolled oats

3⅓ cups unsweetened vanilla almond milk

5 tablespoons plain, unsalted almond butter

2 teaspoons vanilla extract

1 tablespoon plus 2 teaspoons pure maple syrup

3 tablespoons chia seeds

½ cup plus 2 tablespoons sliced almonds

1⅔ cups frozen sweet cherries

Directions:

In a large bowl, mix the oats, almond milk, almond butter, vanilla, maple syrup, and chia seeds until well combined.

Spoon ¾ cup of the oat mixture into each of 5 containers.

Top each serving with 2 tablespoons of almonds and ⅓ cup of cherries.

STORAGE: Store covered containers in the refrigerator for up to 5 days. Overnight oats can be eaten cold or warmed up in the microwave.

Nutrition Info: Total calories: 373; Total fat: 20g; Saturated fat: 1g; Sodium: 121mg; Carbohydrates: 40g; Fiber: 11g; Protein: 13g

Rotisserie Chicken, Baby Kale, Fennel, And Green Apple Salad

Servings: 3

Cooking Time: 15 Minutes

Ingredients:

1 teaspoon olive oil

1 teaspoon chopped garlic

⅔ cup quinoa

1⅓ cups water

1 cooked rotisserie chicken, meat removed and shredded (about 9 ounces)

1 fennel bulb, core and fronds removed, thinly sliced (about 2 cups)

1 small green apple, julienned (about 1½ cups)

8 tablespoons Honey-Lemon Vinaigrette, divided

1 (5-ounce) package baby kale

6 tablespoons walnut pieces

Directions:

Heat the oil over medium heat in a saucepan. Once the oil is shimmering, add the garlic and cook for minute, stirring often so that it doesn't burn.

Add the quinoa and stir a few times. Add the water and turn the heat up to high. Once the water is boiling, cover the pan and turn the heat down to low. Simmer the quinoa for 15 minutes, or until the water is absorbed. Cool.

Place the chicken, fennel, apple, and cooled quinoa in a large bowl. Add 2 tablespoons of the vinaigrette to the bowl and mix to combine.

Divide the baby kale, chicken mixture, and walnuts among 3 containers. Pour 2 tablespoons of the remaining vinaigrette into each of 3 sauce containers.

STORAGE: Store covered containers in the refrigerator for up to days.

Nutrition Info: Total calories: 9; Total fat: 39g; Saturated fat: 6g; Sodium: 727mg; Carbohydrates: 49g; Fiber: 8g; Protein: 29g

Roasted Za'atar Salmon With Peppers And Sweet Potatoes

Servings: 4

Cooking Time: 25 Minutes

Ingredients:

FOR THE VEGGIES

2 large red bell peppers, cut into ½-inch strips

1 pound sweet potatoes, peeled and cut into 1-inch chunks

1 tablespoon olive oil

¼ teaspoon kosher salt

FOR THE SALMON

2¾ teaspoons sesame seeds

2¾ teaspoons dried thyme leaves

2¾ teaspoons sumac

1 pound skinless, boneless salmon fillet, divided into 4 pieces

⅛ teaspoon kosher salt

1 teaspoon olive oil

2 teaspoons freshly squeezed lemon juice

Directions:

TO MAKE THE VEGGIES

Preheat the oven to 4°F.

Place silicone baking mats or parchment paper on two sheet pans.

On the first pan, place the peppers and sweet potatoes. Pour the oil and sprinkle the salt over both and toss to coat. Spread everything out in an even layer. Place the sheet pan in the oven and set a timer for 10 minutes.

TO MAKE THE SALMON

Mix the sesame seeds, thyme, and sumac together in a small bowl to make the za'atar spice mix.

Place the salmon fillets on the second sheet pan. Sprinkle the salt evenly across the fillets. Spread ¼ teaspoon of oil and ½ teaspoon of lemon juice over each piece of salmon.

Pat 2 teaspoons of the za'atar spice mix over each piece of salmon.

When the veggie timer goes off, place the salmon in the oven with the veggies and bake for 10 minutes for salmon that is ½ inch thick and for 15 minutes for salmon that is 1 inch thick. The veggies should be done when the salmon is done cooking.

Place one quarter of the veggies and 1 piece of salmon in each of 4 separate containers.

STORAGE:Store covered containers in the refrigerator for up to 4 days.

Nutrition Info: Total calories: 295; Total fat: 10g; Saturated fat: 2g; Sodium: 249mg; Carbohydrates: 29g; Fiber: 6g; Protein: 25g

Egg Caprese breakfast cups

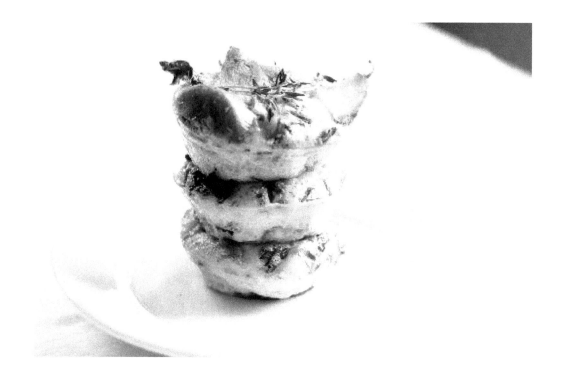

Preparation time: 12 minutes

Cooking time: 17 minutes

Servings: 12

Ingredients:

1/2 tsp garlic powder

4 tbsp basil sliced

12 mozzarella balls

3 cups spinach

12 large eggs

1.25 cups chopped tomatoes

1/2 tsp black pepper

3/4 tsp salt

1-2 tbsp Parmesan cheese grated

balsamic vinegar as required

Directions: In greased muffin cups, make a layer of spinach at the bottom.

Arrange tomatoes, mozzarella, and basil above the spinach layer.

In a mixing bowl, mix salt, cheese, black pepper, garlic powder, and eggs.

Add the egg/cheese mixture in layered muffin cups.

Place the muffin cups for 20 minutes in a preheated oven at 350 degrees.

Drizzle balsamic vinegar and serve.

Nutrition Info: Calories: 141 kcal Fat: 10 g Protein: 11 g Carbs: 1 g Fiber: 1.8 g

Mediterranean mini frittatas

Preparation time: 20 minutes

Cooking time: 25 minutes

Servings: 12

Ingredients:

¼ cup crumbled feta cheese

1 tsp olive oil

1 cup chopped mushrooms

1 cup sliced zucchini

1/3 cup diced red onion

¼ cup chopped Kalamata olives

2 cups spinach

½ tsp dried oregano

½ cup fat-free milk

Six eggs

Black pepper to taste

Directions: Sauté mushrooms, zucchini, and onions for about two minutes in heated oil in a skillet over medium flame.

Mix spinach in the mushroom mixture after lowering the flame. Add oregano and olives.

Cook for two more minutes with occasional stirring. When spinach is done, remove the cooking skillet and set aside.

Mix pepper, eggs, cheese, milk, and sautéed veggies in a bowl.

In an oil muffin pan, pour egg/veggies mixture.

Bake in a preheated oven at 350 degrees for 20 minutes and serve.

Nutrition Info: Calories: 128 kcal Fat: 8 g Protein: 9 g Carbs: 4 g Fiber: 1 g

Caprese avocado toast

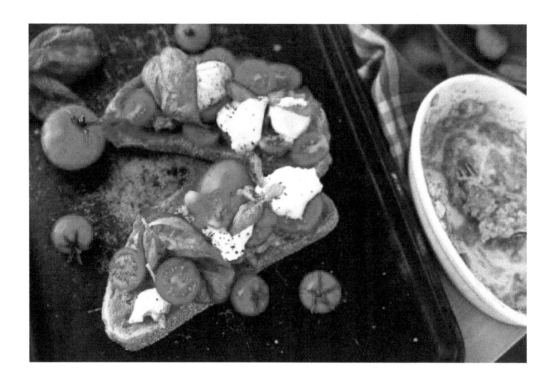

Preparation time: 10 minutes

Cooking time: 0 minute

Servings: 1

Ingredients:

Two avocados

¼ cup chopped basil leaves

2 tsp lemon juice

4 oz sliced mozzarella

Sea salt to taste

Four toasted slices of bread

Black pepper to taste

1 cup halved grape tomatoes

Balsamic glaze for drizzling

Directions: In a bowl, add sliced avocados, salt, lemon juice, and pepper and mix well.

Over medium flame, lightly toast the bread.

Using a knife, spread avocados mixture over bread slices.

Sprinkle salt, basil, cheese, pepper, balsamic glaze, and tomatoes.

Serve and enjoy it.

Nutrition Info: Calories: 338 kcal Fat: 20.4 g Protein: 12.8 g Carbs: 25.8 g Fiber: 9.2 g

Asparagus and mushroom frittata with goat cheese

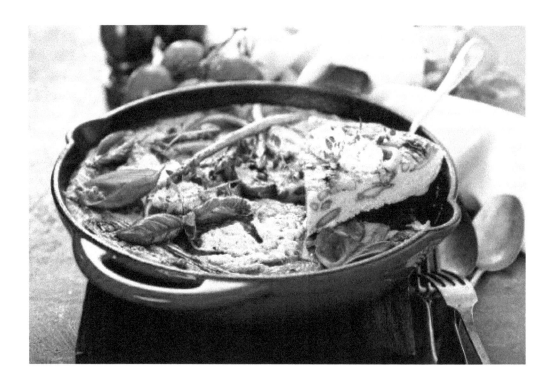

Preparation time: 2 minutes

Cooking time: 8 minutes

Servings: 4

Ingredients:

2 tbsp goat cheese

Two eggs

1pinch of kosher salt

1 tsp of milk

1 tbsp butter

Five trimmed asparagus spears

Three sliced brown mushrooms

1 tbsp chopped green onion

Directions: In a pan, cook mushrooms over medium flame for about three minutes.

Stir in asparagus and cook for two more minutes.

In a bowl, add one tsp of water, eggs, and salt and mix well.

Add the egg mixture to the mushroom mixture, followed by a drizzling of goat cheese and green onions.

Let them cook well until the egg mixture is properly formed.

Shift the pan to the preheated oven and bake for three minutes.

Drizzle cheese and serve.

Nutrition Info: Calories: 331 kcal Fat: 26 g Protein: 20 g Carbs: 7 g Fiber: 2 g

Mediterranean strata

Preparation time: 20 minutes

Cooking time: 55 minutes

Servings: 7

Ingredients:

2 tbsp olive oil

One minced clove garlic

1/2 diced yellow onion

1 lb chicken sausage

1/2 cup halved Kalamata olives

6 cups white bread

1/2 cup chopped sun-dried tomatoes

1/4 cup chopped fresh basil

1/2 cup crumbled feta cheese

Eight eggs

Salt and pepper to taste

2 cups of milk

Red pepper flakes

Directions: Heat butter and oil over medium flame in skillet. Sauté onions for two minutes. Stir in garlic and chicken sausage.

Cook until sausages are done.

Mix olives, cook sausages, onions, sun-dried tomatoes, pepper, bread, garlic, feta cheese, basil, red chili flakes, and salt.

Mix milk and egg in a small bowl and add in sausage mixture.

Pour the sausage mixture into the baking tray.

Bake in preheated oven for 50 minutes and serve after garnishing with basil.

Nutrition Info: Calories: 297 kcal Fat: 9.5 g Protein: 17.9 g Carbs: 36 g Fiber: 3.1 g

Slow cooker Mediterranean egg casserole

Preparation time: 25 minutes

Cooking time: 480 minutes

Servings: 10

Ingredients:

2 oz cut prosciutto

3 cups sliced cremini mushrooms

1 tbsp butter

1/2 chopped red pepper

10 oz chopped spinach

16 oz ORE-IDA Diced Hash Brown Potatoes

1 cup sliced artichoke hearts

8 oz cheddar & Swiss Cheese

1/4 cup chopped sun-dried tomato

4 oz goat cheese

1 tbsp Dijon Mustard

Eight eggs

fresh basil leaves for garnish

2 cups whole milk

Directions: Sauté prosciutto for four minutes in a pan over medium flame. Set aside.

In the same pan, cook bell pepper and mushrooms in the melted butter.

Make layers of potatoes, bell pepper and mushroom mixture, spinach, sundried tomatoes, artichoke hearts, Swiss and cheddar cheese, and goat cheese in the slow cooker.

Mix mustard, milk, salt, eggs, and pepper spread over the veggie's layers in a slow cooker.

Spread prosciutto over the top and cook for about ten minutes on low flame.

Sprinkle basil and serve.

Nutrition Info: Calories: 310 kcal Fat: 19 g Protein: 18 g Carbs: 14 g Fiber: 3 g

Sheet pan eggs and veggies

Preparation time: 10 minutes

Cooking time: 15 minutes

Servings: 6

Ingredients:

One sliced bell pepper (green, red, and orange)

One sliced red onion

Salt to taste

Black pepper to taste

2 tsp za'atar blend,

1 tsp ground cumin and

1 tsp Aleppo chili pepper

Extra virgin olive oil as required

Six eggs

A handful of Chopped fresh parsley

One diced Roma tomato

Crumbled feta cheese

Directions: In a bowl, whisk bell peppers, onions, salt, zaatar, Aleppo chili, cumin, olive oil, and black pepper. Mix well.

Shift the bell pepper mixture over the baking pan.

Bake in a preheated oven at 400 degrees for 15 minutes.

Make holes in baked vegetable mixture and crack one egg in each hole.

Again, bake for eight minutes.

Sprinkle cheese, parsley, and tomatoes and serve.

Nutrition Info: Calories: 111 kcal Fat: 7.3 g Protein: 6.9 g Carbs: 4.5 g Fiber: 1.1 g

Hummus toast

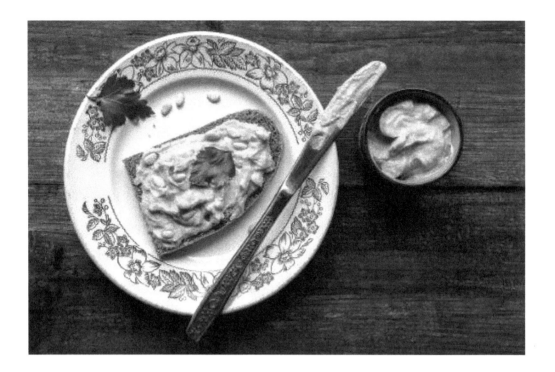

Preparation time: 10 minutes

Cooking time: 0 minute

Servings: 4

Ingredients:

Hummus

Whole-grain bread seeded

Topping option 1

Sprouts

Sliced avocado

Black sesame seeds

Topping option 2

Za'atar spice

Roasted chickpeas

Topping option 3

Sunflower seeds

Pumpkin seeds

Hemp seeds

Sesame seeds

Directions: Spread hummus using a knife over toast and top with any of the topping options given in ingredients and serve.

Nutrition Info: Calories: 300 kcal Fat: 8 g Protein: 10 g Carbs: 24 g Fiber: 7 g

Breakfast egg muffins

Preparation time: 15 minutes

Cooking time: 20 minutes

Servings: 6

Ingredients:

Base

Salt to taste

12 eggs

2 tbsp chopped onion

Black pepper to taste

Tomato spinach mozzarella

Eight sliced cherry tomatoes

1/4 cup chopped spinach

1/4 cup grated mozzarella cheese

Bacon cheddar

1/4 cup grated cheddar cheese

1/4 cup chopped bacon

Garlic mushroom pepper

1/4 cup diced red capsicum

1/4 cup sliced brown mushrooms

1/4 tsp minced garlic powder

1 tbsp chopped parsley

Directions: Mix onions, salt, eggs, and black pepper in a bowl.

Pour egg mixture in muffin cups greased with oil.

Use all three toppings to top each of the muffin cups.

Bake in a preheated oven at 350 degrees for twenty minutes.

Serve and enjoy it.

Nutrition Info: Calories: 82 kcal Fat: 5 g Protein: 6 g Carbs: 1 g Fiber: 1 g

Foul mudammas

Preparation time: 15 minutes

Cooking time: 10 minutes

Servings: 5

Ingredients:

Extra virgin olive oil

Kosher salt to taste

30 oz plain fava beans

1 tsp ground cumin

One lemon juice

1 cup chopped parsley

Two chopped hot peppers

One diced tomato

Two chopped garlic cloves

To serve

Warm pit bread

Green onions

Sliced cucumbers

Sliced tomatoes

Olives

Directions:

Pour half cup of water, salt, beans, and cumin in a pan over medium flame and cook.

When beans are done, mash them using a masher.

Lightly blend garlic, lemon juice, and hot peppers.

Transfer roughly blended hot pepper mixture over mashed beans.

Ass olive oil, parsley, hot pepper slices, and chopped tomatoes and serve with veggies or bread.

Nutrition Info: Calories: 142 kcal Fat: 1 g Protein: 10 g Carbs: 25 g Fiber: 10 g

Tahini banana shakes

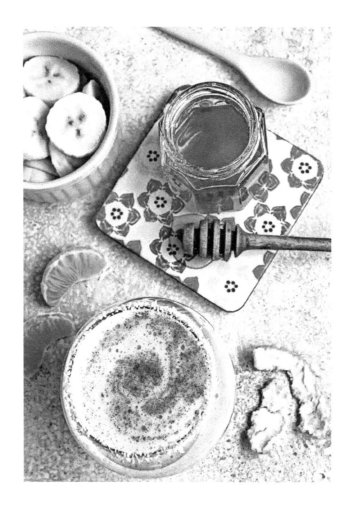

Preparation time: 5 minutes

Cooking time: 0 minute

Servings: 3

Ingredients:

¼ cup ice, crushed

1 ½ cups almond milk

¼ cup tahini

4 Medjool dates

Two sliced bananas

One pinch of ground cinnamon

Directions:

Blend all the ingredients in the blender to obtain a creamy and smooth mixture.

Pour mixture in cups and serve after sprinkling cinnamon over the top.

Nutrition Info: Calories: 299 kcal Fat: 12.4 g Protein: 5.7 g Carbs: 47.7 g Fiber: 5.6 g

Shakshuka

Preparation time: 15 minutes

Cooking time: 20 minutes

Servings: 6

Ingredients:

1 tsp ground cumin

2 tbsp olive oil

One chopped red bell pepper

Six eggs

¼ tsp salt

Three minced cloves garlic

Ground black pepper to taste

2 tbsp tomato paste

½ tsp smoked paprika

¼ tsp red pepper flakes

2 tbsp chopped cilantro for garnish

½ cup feta cheese

One chopped yellow onion

28 oz fire-roasted tomatoes, crushed

Crusty bread for serving

Directions: Heat oil in a skillet over medium flame and cook bell pepper, onions, and salt in it for six minutes with constant stirring.

After six minutes, stir in tomato paste, red pepper flakes, cumin, garlic, and paprika. Cook for another two minutes.

Add crushed tomatoes and cilantro to the onion mixture. Let it simmer.

Reduce the flame and simmer for five minutes.

Use salt and pepper to adjust the flavor.

Crack eggs in small well made at different areas using a spoon. Pour tomato mixture over eggs to help them cook while staying intact.

Bake the skillet in a preheated oven at 375 degrees for 12 minutes.

Garnish with cilantro, flakes, and cheese and serve.

Nutrition Info: Calories: 216 kcal Fat: 12.8 g Protein: 11.2 g Carbs: 16.6 g Fiber: 4.4 g

Simple green juice

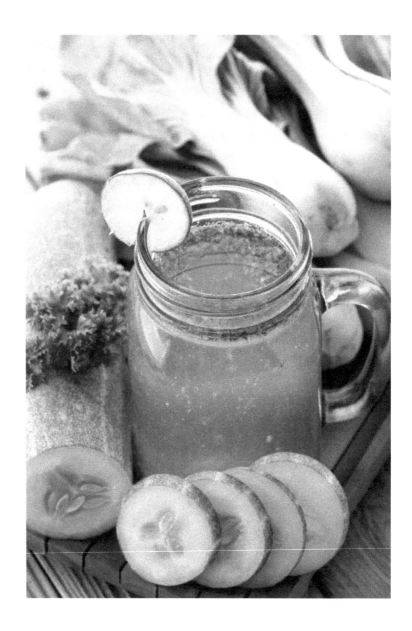

Preparation time: 15 minutes

Cooking time: 0 minute

Servings: 2

Ingredients:

5 oz kale

1 tsp crushed ginger

One apple

Five trimmed celery stalks

½ English cucumber

1 oz parsley

Directions:

Blend all the ingredients in the blender and pour into serving cups.

Nutrition Info: Calories: 92 kcal Fat: 0.8 g Protein: 2.8 g Carbs: 21 g Fiber: 6.2 g

Greek chicken gyro salad

Preparation time: 15 minutes

Cooking time: 7 minutes

Servings: 4

Ingredients:

Chicken

3 tsp dried oregano

2 tbsp olive oil

1 tbsp red wine vinegar

1.25 lb boneless chicken breasts

1 tsp ground black pepper

1 tbsp lemon juice

1 tsp Kosher salt

Salad

1 cup diced English cucumber

6 cups lettuce

1 cup feta cheese diced

1 cup diced tomatoes

1/2 cup diced red onions

1 cup crushed pita chips

Tzatziki Sauce

1 tbsp white wine vinegar

3/4 tsp Kosher salt

8 oz Greek yogurt

One minced clove garlic

2/3 cup grated English cucumber

1 tbsp lemon juice

3/4 tsp ground black pepper

2 tsp dried dill weed

One pinch of sugar

Directions:

Heat oil in a skillet and add chicken, salt, oregano, and black pepper. Cook for five minutes over medium flame.

Reduce the flame to low and add lemon juice and vinegar and simmer for five minutes.

Continue cooking until the chicken is done. Now, the chicken is ready and set aside.

Combine tomatoes, pita chips, chicken, lettuce, cucumber, and onions. Mix and set aside. The salad is ready.

In another bowl, whisk yogurt, cucumber, garlic, lemon juice, vinegar, dill, salt, pepper, and sugar. Mix well. The sauce is ready.

Now, pour the sauce over the salad and serve with cooked chicken.

Nutrition Info: Calories: 737 kcal Fat: 29 g Protein: 64 g Carbs: 54 g Fiber: 6 g

Tuscan tuna and white bean salad

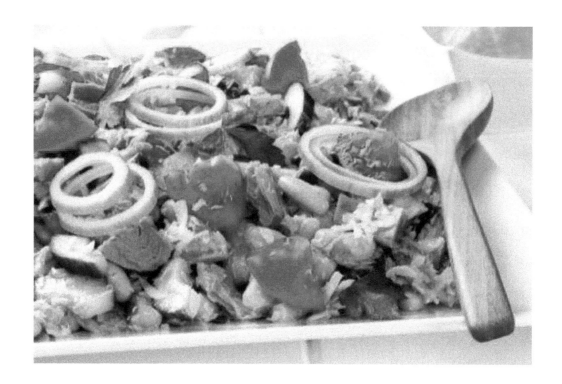

Preparation time: 5 minutes

Cooking time: 0 minute

Servings: 2

Ingredients:

2 tbsp extra virgin olive oil

15 oz cannellini beans

4 cups spinach

5 oz white albacore

1/4 cup sliced olives

1/2 cup diced cherry tomatoes

One sliced red onion

1/2 lemon

Kosher salt to taste

1/4 cup feta cheese

Black pepper to taste

Directions: Combine white beans, olives, lemon juice, arugula, onions, tuna, olive oil, and tomatoes in a mixing bowl.

Sprinkle pepper and salt and feta cheese and serve.

Nutrition Info: Calories: 436 kcal Fat: 22 g Protein: 30 g Carbs: 39 g Fiber: 12 g

Outrageous herbaceous Mediterranean chickpea salad

Preparation time: 20 minutes

Cooking time: 20 minutes

Servings: 4

Ingredients:

1/2 cup chopped celery with leaves

30 oz chickpeas

1.5 cups chopped parsley

1/2 cup chopped onion

3 tbsp olive oil

3 tbsp lemon juice

Two minced cloves garlic

1/2 tsp kosher salt

One chopped red bell pepper

1/2 tsp black pepper

Directions:

Combine bell pepper, onion, chickpeas, celery, and parsley in a mixing bowl.

In another bowl. Mix olive oil, garlic, salt, lemon juice, and pepper.

Pour olive oil mixture over chickpeas mixture and mix well and serve.

Nutrition Info: Calories: 474 kcal Fat: 16 g Protein: 20 g Carbs: 65 g Fiber: 18 g

Avocado Caprese salad

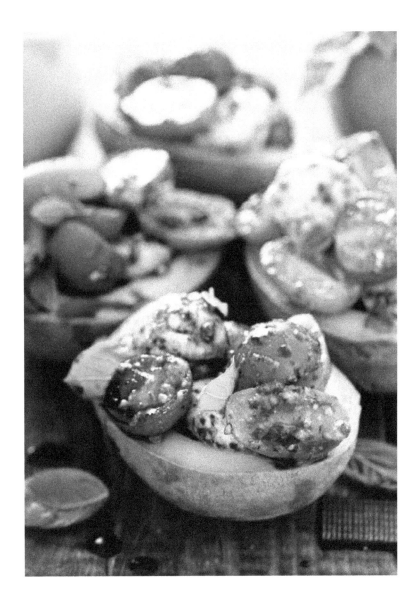

Preparation time: 5 minutes

Cooking time: 0 minute

Servings: 1

Ingredients:

1 cup sliced cherry tomatoes

1/4 cup basil leaves

1/2 cup mozzarella cheese balls

½ avocado

2 tsp extra virgin olive oil

Salt to taste

2 tsp balsamic vinegar

Black pepper to taste

Directions:

In a bowl, combine cheese, tomatoes, avocado, olive oil, salt, basil, vinegar, and black pepper.

Mix well and serve.

Nutrition Info: Calories: 456 kcal Fat: 37 g Protein: 17 g Carbs: 20 g Fiber: 9 g

Citrus shrimp and avocado salad

Preparation time: 5 minutes

Cooking time: 10 minutes

Servings: 3

Ingredients:

1 tbsp olive oil

1/2 cup lemon juice

1 cup of orange juice

1/2 tsp stone house seasoning

3 lb shrimp

2 tbsp chopped parsley

8 cups salad greens

1/2 cup citrus vinaigrette

1/2 sliced red onion

One sliced avocado

Directions:

In a bowl, mix orange juice, stone house seasoning, oil, and lemon juice.

Transfer the bowl mixture to the heated skillet. Cook for five minutes over medium flame.

Stir in shrimps and cook for five more minutes.

Sprinkle parsley and set aside. Citrus shrimps are ready.

Prepare the Citrus Vinaigrette Dressing as per the instruction given on the package.

In a bowl, whisk citrus vinaigrette until it emulsified. Mix salad greens, avocado, shrimps, and onion in a citrus vinaigrette. Serve and enjoy it.

Nutrition Info: Calories: 430 kcal Fat: 21 g Protein: 48 g Carbs: 12 g Fiber: 3 g

Easy couscous with sundried tomato and feta

Preparation time: 12 minutes

Cooking time: minutes

Servings: 6

Ingredients:

1.25 cups dried couscous

1 tsp powdered vegetable stock

1.25 cups boiled water

One chopped garlic clove

14 oz chickpeas

1 tsp coriander powder

½ cup chopped coriander

One chopped onion

½ cup chopped parsley

7 oz sun-dried tomato

One lemon zest

4 oz arugula lettuce

Black pepper

5 tbsp lemon juice

2 oz feta cheese

½ tsp black pepper

Salt to taste

Directions:

In a bowl, combine garlic, chickpeas, stock powder, couscous, and coriander.

Add hot water to the bowl and mix well. Cover the bowl and keep it aside for about five minutes.

Add sun-dried tomatoes, lemon juice, coriander, rocket, pepper, parsley, salt, onions, and lemon zest and toss well.

Sprinkle feta cheese and serve.

Nutrition Info: Calories: 260 kcal Fat: 9.2 g Protein: 10 g Carbs: 39 g Fiber: 5.8 g

Garlicky Swiss chard and chickpeas

Preparation time: 10 minutes

Cooking time: 10 minutes

Servings: 4

Ingredients:

1 cup chopped sundried tomatoes

1 tbsp olive oil Two minced garlic cloves One sliced shallot Two bunches of chopped Swiss chard

15 oz chickpeas One lemon

1/4 cup vegetable broth

Directions:

Cook shallot in heated oil over medium flame until they turned translucent.

After shallots are translucent, stir in garlic and cook for three minutes.

Mix chard and broth and cover, and let it simmer for a few minutes.

Add lemon juice, sundried tomatoes, lemon zest, and chickpeas and mix to combine. Cook for three minutes.

Serve and enjoy.

Nutrition Info: Calories: 519 kcal Fat: 9 g Protein: 14 g Carbs: 87 g Fiber: 10 g

Arugula salad with pesto shrimp, parmesan, and white beans

Preparation time: 35 minutes

Cooking time: 15 minutes

Servings: 3

Ingredients:

4 tbsp olive oil

1/2 lb raw shrimp Two minced cloves garlic

1/4 tsp ground black pepper

1/4 tsp salt

One pinch of red pepper flakes

1/4 cup pesto Genovese 2 cups cherry tomatoes

8 cups Arugula

1/8 cup grated parmesan cheese

1/2 lemon

1/2 cup white beans

Directions: In a mixing bowl, add salt, chili flakes, olive oil, shrimp, and black pepper. Mix well and keep it aside for 30 minutes for enhanced flavor.

Heat olive oil in a skillet over a high flame. Cook shrimps in oil, two minutes from each side.

Lower the flame and stir in tomatoes and garlic. Cook for five more minutes with occasional stirring.

Shift cooked shrimps' mixture in a bowl and mix with pesto.

In a bowl, mix olive oil, arugula, and lemon juice. Add cheese, tomatoes, salt, beans, and black pepper. Mix well.

Serve arugula mixture with cooked shrimps.

Nutrition Info: Calories: 276 kcal Fat: 6.7 g Protein: 30 g Carbs: 23.3 g Fiber: 5.5 g

Cantaloupe and Mozzarella Caprese salad

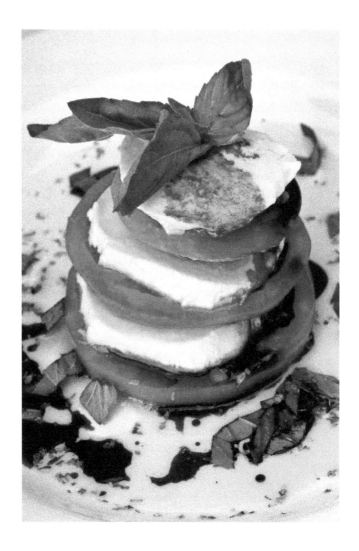

Preparation time: 10 minutes

Cooking time: 0 minute

Servings: 8

Ingredients:

1 tbsp white wine vinegar sliced cantaloupes

Eight shredded prosciutto

8 oz mozzarella balls

¼ cup chopped basil leaves tbsp extra-virgin olive oil

¼ cup chopped mint leaves

Salt to taste

1.5 tbsp honey

Black pepper to taste

Directions: Take cantaloupe balls out of cantaloupe using melon baller and place in a bowl.

Add mozzarella cheese ball, prosciutto, basil, and mint leaves. Mix well.

In another bowl, mix honey, vinegar, and olive oil. Pour the dressing over a cantaloupe mixture and mix well.

Serve and enjoy it.

Nutrition Info: Calories: 232 kcal Fat: 15 g Protein: 10 g Carbs: 17 g Fiber: 2 g

Arugula salad

Preparation time: 5 minutes

Cooking time: 0 minute

Servings: 2

Ingredients:

4 cups arugula tbsp olive oil

1/2 tsp kosher salt tbsp lemon juice

1/2 tsp black pepper

1/4 cup grated parmesan cheese

1 tsp honey

Directions:

Combine honey, black pepper, parmesan cheese, olive oil, salt, arugula, and lemon juice. Toss to coat well.

Serve and enjoy.

Nutrition Info: Calories: 203 kcal Fat: 18 g Protein: 6 g Carbs: 6 g Fiber: 1 g

Mediterranean quinoa salad

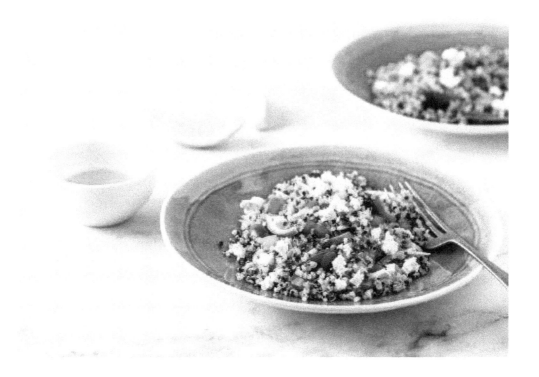

Preparation time: 15 minutes

Cooking time: 0 minute

Servings: 4

Ingredients:

1.5 cups dry quinoa

1/2 tsp kosher salt

1/2 cup extra virgin olive oil

1 tbsp balsamic vinegar minced garlic cloves

1/2 tsp minced basil

1/2 tsp crushed thyme

Black pepper to taste cups arugula

15 oz garbanzo

One package salad savors for toppings

Directions:

In a pot, add water, salt, and quinoa. Cook until quinoa is done. Drain and set aside.

Whisk garlic, pepper, thyme, olive oil, salt, basil, and vinegar in a bowl. The dressing is ready. Keep it aside.

In a big sized bowl, combine salad savor content, arugula, quinoa, and beans.

Pour dressing over the arugula mixture and serve after sprinkling basil over it.

Nutrition Info: Calories: 583 kcal Fat: 33 g Protein: 15 g Carbs: 58 g Fiber: 10 g

Greek pasta salad with cucumber and artichoke hearts

Preparation time: 5 minutes

Cooking time: 0 minute

Servings: 10

Ingredients:

½ cup olive oil

Four minced garlic cloves

1/4 cup white balsamic vinegar tbsp oregano

1 cup crumbled feta cheese

1 tsp ground pepper

15 oz sliced artichoke hearts

1 lb pasta noodles cooked

12 oz roasted and chopped red bell peppers

One sliced English cucumber

8 oz sliced Kalamata olives

¼ sliced red onion

1/3 cup chopped basil leaves

1 tsp kosher salt

Directions: Combine vinegar, oregano, salt, olive oil, garlic, and black pepper in a bowl and mix well. Set aside.

In a big sized bowl, combine olives, onions, cheese, artichoke hearts, cooked pasta, cucumber and bell peppers,

Drizzle dressing over the artichoke hearts mixture and toss to coat. Garnish with feta cheese and basil and serve after half an hour.

Nutrition Info: Calories: 415.43 kcal Fat: 23.15 g Protein: 9.54 g Carbs: 42.54 g Fiber: 4.46 g

Quinoa and kale protein power salad

Preparation time: 5 minutes

Cooking time: 15 minutes

Servings: 5

Ingredients:

One sliced zucchini

½ tbsp extra virgin olive oil

¼ tsp turmeric

¼ tsp cumin

¼ tsp paprika tsp minced garlic,

One pinch of red pepper flakes

½ cup cooked quinoa

Salt to taste

1 cup drained chickpeas

1 cup chopped curly kale

Directions: In a bowl, whisk chili flakes, cumin, paprika, salt, olive oil, garlic, and turmeric. Keep it aside.

Toast quinoa for one minute in olive oil.

Cook toasted quinoa following the instructions given over the package. Set aside.

Sauté garlic, kale, chickpeas, and zucchini in heated olive oil in the same skillet used to toast quinoa.

Cook for a few minutes until the mixture starts to sweat. Sprinkle salt and remove skillet from flame.

In a bowl, combine veggies mixture and quinoa and leave for 10 minutes.

In a skillet, sauté spices in oil for two minutes and add in veggies mixture.

Serve and enjoy.

Nutrition Info: Calories: 106 kcal Fat: 3 g Protein: 5 g Carbs: 16 g Fiber: 4 g

Antipasto salad platter

Preparation time: 20 minutes

Cooking time: 0 minute

Servings: 4

Ingredients:

½ chopped red bell pepper

One chopped garlic clove

12 sliced black olive

¼ cup olive oil

2 tbsp balsamic vinegar

1 tbsp chopped basil

Black pepper to taste

6 oz artichoke hearts

5 oz Italian blend

Salt to taste

1 cup broccoli florets

½ cup sliced onion

Eight strawberry tomatoes 3 oz salami dried 4 oz mozzarella cheese

Directions: In a mixing bowl, mix salt, vinegar, olive oil, black pepper, garlic, and basil. The dressing is ready.

Whisk vinaigrette and salad blend in a bowl.

Transfer the salad blend mixture to a platter and organize all the leftover ingredients on the platter and serve.

Nutrition Info: Calories: 351 kcal Fat: 25.9 g Protein: 16.2 g Carbs: 14.8 g Fiber: 3.8 g

Whole wheat Greek pasta salad

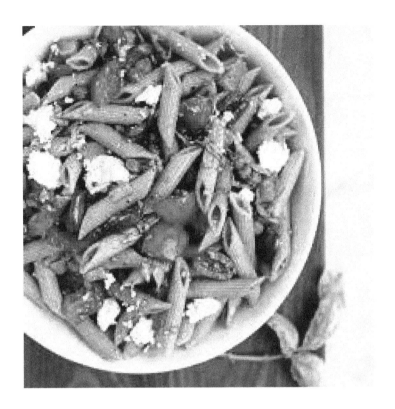

Preparation time: 15 minutes

Cooking time: 0 minute

Servings: 6

Ingredients:

1 lb rotini pasta

One chopped cucumber

1 cup sliced cherry tomatoes

One chopped yellow capsicum

1 cup chopped Kalamata olives

One diced red onion 2 tbsp chopped dill

½ cup feta cheese

Salt to taste

Black pepper to taste

Dressing

2minced garlic cloves

¼ cup olive oil

3tbsp red wine vinegar

½ lemon juice

Salt to taste

½ tsp oregano

Black pepper to taste

Directions: Bring water to boil in a pot. Stir in salt and cook pasta in it until it is done.

Strain pasta and set aside.

Mix Olive oil, vinegar, salt, lemon juice, oregano, pepper, and garlic in a bowl. The dressing is ready.

Combine cooked pasta, cucumber, olives, feta cheese, onions, bell pepper, tomatoes, and dill in a salad serving bowl.

Drizzle dressing over the mixture and toss to coat.

Serve and enjoy it.

Nutrition Info: Calories: 437 kcal Fat: 16 g Protein: 14 g Carbs: 64 g Fiber: 2 g

Tomato and hearts of palm salad

Preparation time: 15 minutes

Cooking time: 0 minute

Servings: 4

Ingredients:

14 oz sliced hearts of palm, diced avocados tbsp lime juice cup sliced grape tomatoes

1/4 cup sliced green onion

1/2 cup chopped cilantro

Salt to taste

Directions:

In a bowl, combine drained and sliced palm hearts, lime juice, tomatoes, avocados, and onions.

Mix salt to adjust the taste.

Sprinkle cilantro to enhance the taste and serve.

Nutrition Info: Calories: 199 kcal Fat: 15 g Protein: 5 g Carbs: 15 g Fiber: 10 g

Quinoa tabbouleh with chickpeas

Preparation time: 20 minutes

Cooking time: 15 minutes

Servings: 8

Ingredients:

1 cup quinoa

2 cups of water

1.5 cups chickpeas cooked cups sliced cherry tomatoescups slicing cucumber

3/4 cups chopped parsley

2/3 cups chopped onions Tbsp chopped mint

Ground Pepper to taste

Dressing

1/3 cups olive oil lemon zest tbsp lemon juice

1.5 tsp minced garlic

¾ tsp salt

Directions: In a bowl, mix lemon juice, salt, oil, lemon zest, and garlic. The dressing is ready.

In a deep pot, add two cups of water, a pinch of salt, and quinoa. Let it boil.

When the water starts boiling, lower the flame to low and cover. Let it simmer for about 15 minutes.

Strain quinoa and set aside to cool down.

In a bowl, combine onions, cucumbers, mint, tomatoes, cooked quinoa, parsley, black pepper, and chickpeas.

Add dressing in quinoa mixture and mix well.

Adjust flavor using black pepper and salt and serve.

Nutrition Info: Calories: 206 kcal Fat: 12 g Protein: 5 g Carbs: 22 g Fiber: 3 g

CPSIA information can be obtained
at www.ICGtesting.com
Printed in the USA
LVHW070803080621
689597LV00023B/2657